Trauma As a Command

Trauma As a Command

Salvatore V. Ambrosino, M.D.

VANTAGE PRESS
New York

FIRST EDITION

Published by Vantage Press, Inc.
516 West 34th Street, New York, New York 10001

Manufactured in the United States of America
ISBN: 0-533-14545-7

Library of Congress Catalog Card No.: 2003090900

0 9 8 7 6 5 4 3 2 1

To my daughter, Barbara Jean Ambrosino, M.D., for her intrepid spirit in her unstinting care of the Other, and also Marie Langone, who was in devoted search for *that* light.

I saw under the sun, that the race is not to the swift, nor the battle to the strong, nor bread to the wise, nor riches to men of understanding, nor fervor to the skillful; but time and chance in all.

—Ecclesiastes: 9:11

Contents

Author's Preface

To live a meaningful life is an act of faith. To live this act of faith, sacrifice must be embraced. To live this sacrifice, a deep commitment of caring must be given to the Other. The Other may be a personal God, or a precious living being, or both.

In this age of quantum physics, there resides an invisible world that is ruled by time and chance. Since he made things mean what he wanted them to mean, Humpty Dumpty seems to have won the field of what is real in life. Relationships of this day appear and disappear as readily as the grin of the Cheshire Cat. The world of this day seems to sit at the table of the Mad Hatter.

A window pane is not a solid substance, although it looks, and feels like a solid—it is a super-cooled liquid. Parallel lines do not meet, but on a sphere, they do meet. Light is neither a particle nor a wave, light is both, depending on the conditions. In the Edison effect, the cathode filaments of a radio tube do not touch the plate, but once these filaments are heated, an electrical current flows from the plates. There was no physical contact! Is life then an illusion bounded by time, chance, and necessity?

Although the atoms of my pen, my brain, and my fingers are made up of the very atoms governed by the stochastic laws of the sub-atomic world, I direct them now to my choices. Now I choose to write this preface to proffer my gift of hope. Now their chaos serves my passion, and this passion directs this world of time and chance to the necessity of my groping for the meaningfulness of love and suffering, the sting that life imparts upon human beings.

My intentionality is served by my willed-action. I challenge no laws. I seek no glory. With this monograph, I have enlisted the service of chaos to help me to sing that in suffering, the human spirit possesses a dimension beyond despair. To live my faith in this hope, I have had to sacrifice much of my finite time, and I have been a witness to the passing of many beautiful days, while I was riveted to this work. I made this sacrifice with no exemptions. And so life must be lived.

When love is not ambivalent and is directed unstintingly to the heart of the Other, and when this love is returned, the circuits of the synaptic self enlist the essences of its deep center that harbors its "I-ness." The confluence of the different aspects of the self, from its biology to its belief systems, becomes a powerful agent to create a companionship with time and chance to enter a transcendental awareness. Chaos can then serve the human epiphanies to bring humanity to the border of goodness. The final leap does need an act of humility in a final surrender to the awe that suffuses life.

This task is not an easy one. The human family has rarely celebrated that we rose out of the primordial soup, and we have achieved much good and much wisdom. We are able to ponder the galaxies billions of light years away with only our brains, minds, and souls. Strangely, this knowledge is not enough, for we also search the heavens for an Other!

Human beings seek that light exploded in Haydn's *The Creation*. Human beings harbor a shard of that divine spark, and with this little light, they seem to look homeward as if they were angels trying to find their way back to their birthplace.

Perhaps all music tries to reach that grander light. Perhaps when all the music of the human soul has been played, then all of humanity will have found rest and peace.

Trauma is a command to find that light!

We shall not cease from exploration.
And the end of all our exploring
Will be to arrive where we started
And know the place for the first time.
T. S. Eliot, *Four Quartets,* "Little Gidding, V"

Author's Note

For many years I spoke of trauma as a command. As a resident in psychiatry, I would apply this principle. As the years wore on, I was not sure of its origin. I thank my daughter, Antoinette Ambrosino Wyszynski, M.D., who traced it to its source.

Otto Sperling, "The Interpretation of Trauma as a Command," *Psychoanalytic Journal.* 19:382 (1950).

Men's curiosity searches past and future
And clings to that dimension. But to apprehend
The point of intersection of the timeless
With time, is an occupation for a saint.

T. S. Eliot *Four Quartets;* "The Dry Salvages, V"

Acknowledgments

I would like to thank all my teachers who taught me so well in neuro-psychiatry at Bellevue Hospital (NYU). Sam Wortis, M.D.; Morris Hermm, M.D.; Marvin Stern, M.D.; John Frosch, M.D.; Gustav Bychowski, M.D.; Arthur Zitrin, M.D.; Morris Bender, M.D.; Archer Silver, M.D.; Lauretta Bender, M.D.; and David Wechsler, Ph.D.

The patience and guidance of my friends who put this monograph together:
Patty Wolff, Jacqueline Leone, Barbara Stagnitta, Jim Pinto, Tony Oliviero, Michael Burgio, Sandy Bordi, John Mignosa, Frank Cottone, Michael Fenton, and Maria Alessi—I thank you.

My special thanks to Ambassador Gargano who took time out of his heavy schedule to review this work.

I would also like to thank Dr. Robert Cancro, Chairman of the Department of Psychiatry at NYU School of Medicine for his review of this monograph.

And as always, for my good wife, who suffers through all the stages of my fulminating ideas, thank you.

—God Bless

Introduction

Trauma As a Command is a poignant and pivotal body of work on trauma. This monograph provides important guidance for those who suffer "inconsolable losses." In this monograph I found great comfort and hope to deal with the tragedy of the Twin Towers.

September 11, 2001 began as any other day. The sun's rays initiated their descent on our tallest skyscrapers towards the city's streets. Meanwhile, our citizens embarked upon their ascent into morning routines. The street vendors arrived in preparation for their most loyal customers. "Closed" signs were changed to "open." Through our tunnels, over our bridges, on our buses, and out of our underground labyrinth, the streets became alive with the hustle and bustle of commuters. As we all know too well, life would change drastically within minutes.

The events that occurred that Tuesday morning changed our lives and will continue to challenge all generations. This incomprehensible tragedy resulted in the loss of thousands of lives, treasured buildings, cherished beliefs, and a sense of safety. As a nation, we shared fear, shock, panic, grief, despair, anger, frustration, and even the need to take action. In the days, and now months that have followed, we have found that in addition to these shared reactions, we have all been privately affected by this event.

Through the blanket of dust covering our streets and a mass escape of business men and women, heroes rose out of the rubble and continue to emerge in expected and unexpected places. From our firefighters, our police officers, and our emergency workers, who traveled to the scene and remained behind, to the mother comforting her family from the inevitable news, heroes were made.

Through projecting hope, confidence, and optimism, we can help ourselves along with others. No one ever expected such an event to happen. This tragedy shook our streets and our people, physically and emotionally. Therefore September 11th evoked an unthinkable trauma to the nation's children and adults. As each of us tries to grasp the events of that day, a wide variety of thoughts, emotions, and symptoms are understandable responses to traumatic events.

Like Fritz Koenig's *The Sphere* that once graced the Trade Center's plaza, we have all been marked forever by the destruction. However, like the new meaning of hope and honor we have placed on this embattled sculpture, we must also create new hope and meaning for ourselves. It is also imperative that we realize the need for healing. We must try to find value and grow from this experience.

Since this most heinous attack ever on American soil, I do not think I have completed one day without asking myself why such an event happened and why so many of our loved ones were lost. I do not think I will ever know the answers to these questions, nor will many of us. But we can, and will, find solace in ourselves and others.

Through the spirits and inspiring tales of our heroes, we will forge past this great tragedy with its pain and grief that followed. We will excel in the rebuilding and memorializing of our loved ones' courageous deeds as well as our own. There is no single, right reaction to the events of September 11th. The people lost forever were husbands and wives, sons and daughters, friends and colleagues. They were our valued loved ones. In dealing with trauma, our inner self and mental state must guide us towards managing us to rise above our grief. To go within ourselves, to the best of our deeper self, will help us to respond to this trauma as a command to transcend our pain and strengthen ourselves and America.

—Ambassador Charles Gargano
Chairman, Empire State Development Corporation

Trauma As a Command

A Daunting Challenge

What life have you if you have not life together?
There is no life that is not in community
And no community not lived in praise of God.
—T. S. Eliot, *The Rock*

Trauma is a wound. In Medicine, a wound is an injury to living tissue caused by an outside, or a foreign agent. In this monograph, the wound will be considered to be a mental one, a psychic trauma. The wound will be taken to be a loss, an inconsolable loss with no secondary gains. Such loss will be referred to as *real* loss.

The psychic trauma will be examined as a threat to the wholeness or integrity of the person, the Self. The psychic effect will be taken as a possible threat to the continuity of the Self. The wound or trauma will be a *real* loss that is immediate, anticipated or imagined. For example, a soldier in combat may anticipate the loss of a limb, or he may imagine its loss. His psychic reaction to the loss is the "wound." In any case, the pain is real. Sometimes the loss will serve a purpose, a secondary gain, as in war when a loss will remove a soldier from combat.

Real loss, or its threat, carries the feeling that a permanent change in the Self will occur. When a valued object, limb or a loved one, is gone, the feeling that once was attached to the object seems to float through the air like a ghost looking for a new attachment. That affective detachment is the psychic wound. The psychic response can manifest itself in a number of ways.

Psychic Responses to Trauma

In *real* Loss, the detached affect makes demands upon the psyche to be reintegrated with the Self. These responses can be merely adaptive, or creative, depending upon the maturity of the Self:

1. The sweet lemon, or the sour grape—this is the rationalization that the object lost was not necessary; its value is purposely diminished to diminish its affective impact.
2. Denial—"nothing happened; nothing has been lost," what was once conscious, is out of awareness.
3. Working through—what was lost, and its meaning is examined at many levels of consciousness and feeling reactions, i.e., from dreams to waking life.
4. Magical undoing—rituals are established to undo the death, e.g., contact with the dead through channeling or séances, or excessive mourning.
5. Shifting of responsibility—to diminish the impact of possible guilt experienced vulnerability, the loss is ascribed to a more powerful object, e.g., God, or a parent.
6. Surrender of the self to the offending, or more powerful agent, e.g., children playing "doctor."

7. Creative reintegration—to keep in touch with the feelings of the real loss, either by holding them in abeyance until a better day, or the use of a linking object (an object associated with what was lost) e.g., a comb, a watch. The less ambivalent the relationship, the less pathological the linking.

In the Post Traumatic Stress Syndrome, what is most outstanding is the panic that causes a suffering, which for a long time resists all reason, consolation, and reassurance. Not only is the person easily startled, but any exposure to the traumatic event could precipitate a panic reaction. Consequently, people avoid any resemblance to the noxious experience; in fact, the dreams in this condition are nightmares in which the person re-experiences the traumatic event.

Underlying this reaction to trauma is the utter helplessness of the person, and the urgent need to decrease the sense of helplessness. This sense can be ameliorated with the use of medication, and with a dependability of the Other, namely the psychiatrist. Amazing to behold is the improvement that can take place, when the offending agent no longer sets off an anxiety attack or the panic. What is of interest is that after clinical recovery very few persons ever "grow" from the experience, that is their suffering does not bring them to a new experience of themselves, or to the Other. There is no enlarged vista either of personalization or humanization, i.e., no clearer definition of the Self, or giving of oneself to another.

Objects lost can be things, physical or psychic of the Self, or of the Other. The response is determined by affects, values, and the state of the historical process. The feeling attached to a lost object is the affective component, i.e., how important the watch was, or how important was one's arm, or how important self-esteem was held, or how important a mother was. That affective quality carries a value, and this value must be much more than a magical dependent one for magical dependency carries too much ambivalence for its persistence. Dealing with loss depends upon the historical process that has characterized an individual's development. The confrontation with trauma can lead to sudden helplessness, the numbness of depersonalization, momentary disorganization, or despair. The confrontation can also produce a yearning to be in touch with the lost object, or to retrieve one's own history. These responses play a large role in the experience of trauma. The chronic experience or trauma can numb the whole process of growth with helplessness as a permanent feature.

In *real* loss, there is then a whole spectrum of responses within the phenomenology noted above. In *real* loss, especially of a loved one, a modicum of regret, shock, disbelief, ambivalence (always lingering love/resentment), despair, and a desire for return is almost always there. Beyond narcissism (self-love), and masochism (self-defeat), human beings shroud themselves in a cloak of invincibility: many soldiers had the feeling in combat, "I will not be killed!" Like a baseball player in a batting slump, all kinds of magical rituals are used to turn the tide of the "bad" luck. Do not many carry a "lucky" rabbit's paw of one kind or another to have good fortune shine upon them? Often I wonder whether the post burial collation is not an example of this magical undoing, a yearning to maintain contact with the lost one. The process of taking in, introjection, can play a large role in the human need to keep the valued person alive within the Self, not only out of love, but also for spiritual strength. Among Roman Catholics the introjection of communion is much more than a ritual of identification. For them the belief is that a promise has been kept, and has perpetuated a relationship with a transcendental Other.

Command, the Self, Reality, and the Deep Center

The word "command" is derived from the Latin *commandare* (to commit to one's charge, or give an authority to issue an order). In this monograph, "command" is used as a hovering imperative, a kind of angel in the whirlwind, who beckons choice beyond the Self. In a very realistic example, albeit a common one, on my first day in the army, my First Sergeant, with his six stripes surrounding a diamond, brought his nose to my own and succinctly announced to me in a stentorian voice that henceforth, he was my mother. In a forceful tone, he commanded me to remember that there were only two ways of doing things: his way and no other way! This is a concrete example of trauma as a command: I was eighteen years old, and to be eligible for medical school one day, I would need the record of a good soldier—no dishonorable discharge. My sergeant's exhortation chiseled my focus that I was now in the Army, and indeed his beckoning was a command to seek out an Ego Ideal that would warrant me survival in a war and the reward of an honorable discharge for peacetime.

During my first Mass in the Service, our army chaplain gave us a reminder that those who came into the Service with sincerity, honesty, and cooperation would leave the Army "better men." He suggested that the horrendous experience of war could be a catalyst to bring out the best of us. His command was that of an angel of another kind—find the best of yourselves to serve a common cause that was above your own.

In both examples, there was no sense of helplessness, no wounds, no *real* losses, except perhaps that of the loss of self-esteem and the ostracism that could come with a poor service record. In this monograph, I refer to more devastating trauma that befell people, overwhelming experiences that could have left people bereft and disoriented. I want to study those persons who were able to rise above a devastated state. I want to examine those few who responded to the trauma of *real* loss with a raised consciousness and gathered themselves to the synthesis of a new hope. For these few, the traumatic event rendered their spirits almost indomitable. In such cases, the traumatic event is almost taken as a challenge, not to be lost in the space of self-pity and easy rationalization, but to rise above the suffering.

In the ordinary sense, command carries an imperative mood, an imperious urging on, for example, "Come here," with the pronoun "you" understood. In this monograph, the experienced trauma is taken as a clarion sounding of the imperative mood, that is, as an *active* call to action. If outside forces can cause psychic disruption with the loss of Self-connectedness, perhaps the wound can be healed by a return to the inner world of the psyche, beyond external chaos to real connections of the deep Self. Then affects and ideas would be appropriate to the Self and could be directed with humility to the "wounds" of the others. Disruption is fostered by narcissism and masochism which makes integration of the Self impossible. Narcissism speaks only of self-caring and masochism speaks only of self-defeat. As my chaplain implied, one must look within the largess of oneself to meet the stress of life. To share this largess within depends on the ability to live in the mysterious paradox that to give of oneself is to heal oneself. Life must become much more of "what can I know?"; much more of "what can I hope for?"; and certainly "what might I do?" Such transformation can only take place when there is a willingness to share one's deeper core with the Other!

Before proceeding, I would like to offer some clarification of the Self and of reality. As pointed out in one of my previous publications, I take the Self to be "the whole person; body, mind, and soul!" I also pointed out that the part of the Self that analyzes and executes the action is the Ego. I consider the Ego to be made of boundaries:

> The *outer one* is made of the special senses, such as vision, smell, hearing, taste, and position in space, while the *inner one* is made up of attitudes, beliefs and ethical-moral values.

Human beings incorporate the world through the process of introjection. Character is that measure of the Self that houses its ethical-moral values, and its stability is formed by the consistency of moral and ethical traits that mark the person. The personality is the organized totality of the Self's character traits, attitudes, and habits and how that personality responds affectively and cognitively to create behavior. While the Self responds to "unconscious," preconscious, and conscious reality, it is temperament that shapes the reaction of the total Self to the world. "Unconscious" reality means out of the awareness of intentionality, but retrievable through daydreams, dreams, slips of the tongue, and the quality of our behavior. Preconscious reality is readily retrievable once focused upon, e.g., "What is your birthday?" Conscious reality is what is there now in one's focus. Temperament is constitutional and inherited and "governs the mode of emotional response." Temperament involves the reactivity of the nervous system, and this is inherited. The body type is part of this inheritance. The temperaments are nervous (anxious), cheerful (sanguine), gloomy (saturnine), stolid (phlegmatic), unhappy or irritable (dysphoric), hypercharged (hypomanic), impulsive (hyperkinetic).

While temperament shapes the responses, the governing brake on the action is both social and universal or global consciousness. Consciousness is much more than neurological awareness, for it contains one's viewpoint of life and often is tacit. Consciousness is not an allegory, for its level of experience determines its boundaries. In this way, social guilt yields to the higher guilt, which is an error in every culture e.g., killing someone because they are different. Consciousness is that state of being in which an organism can look upon itself in reflection, and through an established intentionality, direct its choices. The awareness that all human beings are connected by Melville's "monkey-rope," what affects one, also affects the other.[1] Beyond cultural practice, there is then Conscience with its global Consciousness: a non-wearing eyeglass culture has no right to vote death to those who do wear eyeglasses. The majority may rule, but they could be wrong in a consciousness beyond their culture.

Reality is much more than an act or a process of learning, as in a valid syllogism: all men are mortal: John is a man, therefore John is mortal. Human experience and its perceptions include affects, (emotional responses). Human beings relate with affects to the perceived world hopefully in an appropriate manner. For example, on a sunny day, the person who cannot experience its brightness, or the one who moves about in a mechanical, robotic way is depersonalized; but those who experience the world as not being real have become derealized.

When the affective investment of the Self in the outside world is diminished, the *sense* of reality has changed despite its cognitive appreciation. When a person is not able to relate to another, whether for psychological or temperamental reasons, the *relationship* with reality has been altered. Reality is then made up of an act of knowing, a sense of knowing, and a relationship to what is known. In its final act, the SELF is governed not only by social and global consciousness, but also by the North Star of the Self, the Ego Ideal. This Ego Ideal is a derivative of the social consciousness, and is formed by looking up to the life of an admired person followed by the identification with, and introjection of the admired qualities to create the deep center of one's Self. As Polonius said to his son Laertes:

This above all,—
To thine own self be true
And it must follow as the night the day,
Thou canst not then be false to any man.

(*Hamlet,* 1.3.78-81)[2]

A whole person develops a social consciousness, which becomes one with global consciousness. This may represent the state of being of St. Paul's ideal of Caritas, or even Beethoven's "*Diesen Kuss der ganzen Welt*" (This kiss for all the world).

The workhorse for the Self is the Ego, that in trying to fulfill its Ideal must like itself, and it is this feeling that prompts the injunction "to love thy neighbor as thyself."

The Ego maintains its wholeness by suffusing itself with a Self-caring and a Self-liking, only to be completed in radiating this Self-love to alight upon the Other. Ego wholeness is necessary to insure an accurate perception of the world and its reality. In giving to the other, the Self completes itself, and this connection is achieved through the Ego. For this reason, the Ego is taken to assist in three spheres of influence to maintain its wholeness, which is reflected in the integrity of the Self. These Ego Spheres are:

1. The Sphere of *experiencing,* or its history,
2. The Sphere of *differentiation,* so that free choices and action belong to the Ego itself, and none other, and
3. The Sphere of *affective resolution,* so that the feelings for the other reflect the consistency of the Self.

The wholeness of the Ego is reflected in the appropriate consistency of what it thinks, feels, and acts upon. At first in a parochial consciousness, and later in its historical process to a global consciousness. Human beings must get to know their freedom of thought and its price,

Know then thyself, presume not God to scan;
The proper study of mankind is Man.

(*Essay on Man,* 2.1–2)[3]

Up to this point, I have been defining the psychological basis that will help a person to respond to trauma in a creative way. Later I shall refer to those transitional human beings who move from a deep center, from a "germinal higher part," those whose experiences can go "beyond the ego consciousness but which nevertheless affects consciousness." Those individuals who are able to go "beyond the ego-centered condition," and in their selflessness, they become themselves creative powers.

T. S. Eliot spoke of the timeless moment, the point of interaction of the timeless with time. "To go beyond the Psychology of the equivalent, felt as death: But it is a dying to be reborn, reborn in depth."[4]

At the moment which is not of action or inaction
You can receive this: "on whatever sphere of being
The mind of a man may be intent
At the time of death"—that is the one action
(And the time of death is every moment)
Which shall fructify in the lives of others:
And do not think of the fruit of action.
Fare forward.

(T. S. Eliot, *Four Quartets* "The Dry Salvages")[5]

These transitional creatures live at that "point of interaction" and their "sphere of being" is a daily "dying to be reborn" in sacrifice. They become the conduits "for the creative power."

In *The Swelling Tide,* I spoke of these transitional beings who transform the focus of life from mere adaptation to a "pursuit of truth and the expansion of consciousness." [6] For them "the path, the way, is the goal!" These are those who "bring their passion of inner faith and conviction into the precarious experience of their commitment." From their deep center, they surrender their Ego boundaries, and complete themselves, center to center, with and in the Other.

Sir John Eccles spoke of the "liaison Brain"[7] as that transitional zone that opens the brain to "mental influences."[8] Perhaps, metaphors, myths, and rituals stew in that deep center of those transitional beings, wherein Bohr felt that "materialism and spiritualism . . . are two aspects of the same thing."[9] Perhaps from this deep center, deaf Beethoven composed his great *Missa Solemnis.* Perhaps, all art is beyond utility and defines the timeless dimension, wherein transformations of crosses of destruction become crucifixes of hope. Perhaps, all art stews in the consciousness of the deep center, that can only complete itself in the center of the other. Perhaps, art is all about those musical notes that we do not hear, but whose effects upon human hearts confirm their existence. Perhaps, the unseen keeps us in orbit around our precious Sun. Perhaps these transitional beings do not look to things purely in a rational way, but from their own within. The interpretation of poetry renders it banal because poetry is understood in the heart. Perhaps, that is why today "nothing" has become "something" for scientists.

The Sphere of Ego Experiencing

When trauma befalls a person, the total Self experiences its impact, and this occurs at a particular time of its *process* of maturation. The maturity of the Ego at the time of the traumatic impact will determine much of the reaction of the Self:

a. If the trauma were to occur at the time when the Ego is poorly differentiated, there could be a total collapse of the Self manifested by
   i. strict denial—"nothing is wrong—nothing happened," or
   ii. complete surrender—"I'm too weak"
b. If the Ego were to be early in its development, the person may identify with the traumatic agent or remain fixated at that stage of development, or
c. If the trauma were to occur later in development, after relationships have been formed, the person might choose to experience *less* of himself, or of the world, resulting in derealization or depersonalization and become numb to the world or to the Self.
d. If the Ego were fairly well-differentiated, retreat or regression may take place in the service of Self.

How the Ego reacts to a trauma then depends on the suddenness of the trauma and how capable the Ego may be to assimilate the traumatic impact. The state of Ego preparation depends upon a number of factors:

1. Temperament,
2. differentiation of the Ego,
3. the development of a deep center for the Self,
4. family experience, and
5. the personal mark of the individual to deal with reality.

As an example, if a four-year-old boy lost his father who had been chronically ill and if the child had been loved by his father, and if his mother were of a sanguine temperament, the child would fare much better than a similar child left to a depressive, fault-finding mother, especially if she were an alcoholic. The temperament of the affected person would be very important: the child of the happier, non-fault-finding person would fare much better than the child of the complaining one.

In sudden loss, the Ego does not have much time to make adjustments to the altered experience. In slow moving traumatic experiences, the Ego has an opportunity to employ defense mechanisms from minimization to rationalization to soften the blow of loss. The familial milieu with its affectivity, the quality of its emotional responses and its values is important. What is also crucial in meeting traumatic insults is the degree to which the Ego has been able to distinguish its feelings, strengths, and actions from the Other with a sense of responsibility for its own actions. The development of an integrated deep center of the Self with an ability to love and to be loved and to know right from wrong is most important. This Sphere of

Ego experiencing depends then on the close operation of an Ego free of conflict and splits in the service of a responsible, deep-centered Self.

Anne Frank was a sensitive, sanguine personality who had found refuge in her family, her music, and her diary. She seemed to have a clear idea of who she was, but once she lost her sister, her will to survive was compromised. The loss overwhelmed her, and she lacked the strength to go on. Her dependence upon her sister weakened her Ego's ability to survive such a loss. In traumatic experiences, a well-differentiated Ego is unfettered to other beings, such an Ego is able to exercise an appropriate adjustment when confronted with the need to make a free choice of altered attitude to preserve the Self.

In Freud's case of Anna O., the conflict of ambivalent feelings in the care of her sick father was so repressed that she developed a myriad of symptoms: blindness, loss of her voice, threatened starvation, and limb "paralysis."[10] The trauma experienced was her loss of freedom, and being unable to make an appropriate choice for her Self, her Ego split in its execution and directed her affective reactions into her body, somatization. In this way her choice was neutralized, if only for the moment.

I had a patient who had been a soldier in the Korean War. He had been a happy-go-lucky wise-cracking, typical GI, who presented himself with a bravado that seemed to indicate that he did not spend much time in thought about his actions. His life was all here and now. He had a very close buddy with whom he spent much time. They had been together in a number of combat engagements. One day their platoon had to attack an enemy hill. As they proceeded up the hill in the beginning engagement, my patient said to his buddy in his typical style, "Let's go and get some gooks." He proceeded up the hill, only to find himself alone. Subsequently, he found his buddy dead at the bottom of the hill with a bullet hole between his eyes.

Immediately upon seeing his buddy, he dropped to the ground and could not move his legs—he was "paralyzed." He slowly recovered from his paralysis, but for years after the war, he had suffered severe anxiety attacks. Later, in an Amytal interview ("truth serum"), he was able to remember that, at the very time when he had seen his buddy dead for a brief moment, he silently said to himself: "better you than me." The sudden loss fused with his own deep fear about combat and the reality that he too could be killed, was so traumatic that his Ego was overwhelmed by the reality of his vulnerability in a chanceful world. He was not prepared to deal with his own intense desire to live.

Another patient was a U. S. Marine in WWII. He had held off a Japanese night attack on his position in a South Pacific battle. The next morning many dead Japanese soldiers lay before his position. With his machine gun, he had prevented the enemy to enfilade the Marine position. He had expected, if not a commendation, praise from his company commander. Upon seeing what the marine had done, the captain cynically remarked "not bad for a wop." The marine was an Italian-American. Not only was he not commended, but he was also greeted by this pejorative expletive. The marine awakened in an aid station: he had "blanked out," for, in an altered consciousness, he tried to kill his officer. Later it was learned that his father was never pleased with any of his achievements and never praised him. The terror of combat was not the trauma, but the re-experienced loss of self-esteem was the trauma, which overwhelmed his Ego and split his consciousness.

In the Sphere of Ego Experiencing, defense mechanisms are "unconscious" ways for the Ego to deal with conflict. Repression and denial are defense mechanisms, and share some common psychic ground. Both manage to postpone problems for the moment, and create "psychic debts," which, unredeemed by the Ego, their imperative nature will affect the wholeness of the Ego, its mind, body, or both. In the cases of Anna O. and the Korean veteran, there was "paralysis," and for Anne Frank and the marine, an altered consciousness. None of the individuals presented was prepared for the trauma that befell them, and they did not "grow from their experiences."

Crucial differences exist, however, between denial and repression. In children, denial is almost "pure" in that it may not occur with other defense mechanisms. Children react to the world with behavior and attitude, so that conceptualizations are not available from them. Their behavior and their attitudes must be deciphered. For this reason, when children are confronted with the overwhelming trauma of loss, they seem not to react. In their budding Ego, unable to cope with the whole meaning of loss, they seem to deny the traumatizing event, and under the pressure of bewilderment, born of cognitive immaturity and intensive affective pain, they deny the loss despite their intuitive grasp of things. They seem to split the event: the sighted venomous cobra is regarded to be that of a harmless garden variety.

In denial there seems to be an awareness of the traumatic event, but the event is minimized, or isolated. For example, traumatized by a redheaded father, followed by denial, can eventuate in the drowning of a child if he were to wave off a redheaded lifeguard who is trying to save him. Unable to fit the "blame" onto the father, the child then blames all redheaded people, and years later in denial of the reality, his feelings for his father are not addressed and the child drowns. Relatedness to the world can be affected by such denial, because the Ego does not relate either to the Self in a full measure, resulting in the numbness of depersonalization, or to the outside world in full radiance causing a derealization. The Self and the world are perceived in *cognitive* reality, but the *sense* of reality is fogged, and the *relationship* with the outside world becomes numbed and matter-of-fact. The Self is consequently "dismembered" and sees a world without color. Once I had a patient who felt that her limbs extended to the fenders of the car, her head on its roof, and her back was at the rear of the car. In the same vein, another patient once remarked, "I was whittled down to a toothpick."

Denial is almost a complete break with the offending reality, whereas in repression, there seems to be a remnant Ego need to bring the conflict to the surface of full consciousness. In repression, there are escapes from the "unconscious" in slips of the tongue, daydreams, dreams, fantasies, memories, "mistakes," and even in perverted acts. Repression has a delay factor and involves much more the within of the person (desires, thoughts, feelings, memories). Denial is much more related to a disavowal of external reality.

Traumatic events are external to the Self, but the reactions to the event occur within the Self, affecting both mind and body. These reactions are discharged through the sphere of the experiencing Ego. The best preparation for life is the wholeness or the integrity of the Self whereby one's thoughts, feelings, and actions are discharged in an appropriate, consistent, and harmonious manner. No splits. Most traumatic events take place without warning, and for this reason, the pre-traumatic wholeness of the Self is so crucial.

An exception to this observation applies to the victims of the Holocaust of WWII. The unthinkable massiveness of suffering of those people is beyond comprehension. They were so deprived of everyday needs, of all hope of a future. Worst of all, the deeper parts of their Self were deprived of those whom they loved, and these deeper parts held no hope to be able to help their loved ones, or themselves. Those victims were immersed in steel containers with no light and no exits. In order to understand how they fared with such unimaginable hopelessness with such loss of freedom, one would have to establish a whole new approach to the problem of trauma and its effects upon the souls of people. Victor Frankl gives us such insight.

Frankl emphasized that emphasis on everyday survival eventuated in becoming one of the enemy. Living for oneself was a form of death. He stressed, however, that to live beyond mere survival, one had to recognize what the external reality was, remain true to what one believed in and what one loved, and then to exercise one's last choice in that freedom despite painful, overwhelming circumstances.

As noted, a traumatic event etches itself into the memory system, and its manifestations are panic attacks, startled reactions and nightmares. Indeed, the brain becomes involved. These experiences indicate that the Sphere of Ego experiencing has underlying consequences in the nervous system. One must wonder whether those who respond to a trauma as a command to a higher integration of the Self possess a special type of brain.

The Sphere of Ego Differentiation

To cope with traumatic experiences, a person must invest much thoughtful and emotional energy to counter the impact of the trauma. Despite the absence of physical wounds, the body is subject to great pressures that can leave scars. While anxiety is a psychic state of anticipation, tension is a body response of this continuous preparedness. The counter movements to the trauma can involve any of the defense mechanisms. To be remembered is that those mechanisms are out of Ego awareness ("unconscious") and are brought into play whenever this psyche is confronted with difficult conflicts. As mentioned, denial or repression can follow, but there can also be the minimization of *isolation,* the extra work of *over-compensation,* the bitter being made sweet of *rationalization,* the retreat of *regression* to happier times, and the *Self-service of regression* in service of the Ego.

One may also confront directly the traumatic event. To deal with traumatic events in such a manner, a "conflict-free" Ego would be necessary so that it could be free of internal contradictory demands and conflicts. Only in this way could the perception of external happenings be clear, and therefore not overwhelm. A "free" Ego is one then that has been differentiated from the demands of the outside world and inner world objects. No foreign bodies displace the values of the Self. Such an Ego has evolved from a deep center of nonambivalent caring. In this deep center, the cardinal virtues of honesty, justice, humility, and fortitude reside.

C. S. Lewis points out that the cardinal values are "pivotal" in how a person lives his life. Honesty includes common sense and fair play: To say it as it is, and to do it as it is. This idea includes the justice to be consistent and fair-minded. Humility encompasses the awareness that one is not all powerful; patience and openness of mind are its benchmarks. Fortitude is that courage to face what lies before one, and to persist in one's choices, albeit however unpopular or difficult. The Self through its Ego deals with the rightness or wrongness of its acts, its morality. Making choices both in the social sphere of the Super-ego and the global sphere of the Conscience requires judgments that depend on:

1. The wholeness of the Self,
2. The relationship between the Self and the Other,
3. The personal belief system of what force brought life to earth,
4. The personal concept of where they belong in the universe.

In order for this world to happen, there must be responsible, free choice emanating from a deep center of the Self in which there reside the cardinal virtues and a willingness to give from the Self. A conflict-free Ego therefore does not deny what looms before it. With clear vision it will act in a virtuous way. With such an Ego structure, if regression were to take place, it would be a temporary way station in which a person gathers one's thoughts and feelings before acting on what must be done. Such an action requires wholeness and harmony within the Self and a feeling of connectedness to the outside world. A well-differentiated Ego has described itself free to itself, and paradoxically connected to the world outside. A well-differentiated Ego is resilient and rarely loses its focus on its deep center and on the center of the Other. Psychic retreats or regressions can take place, but in such a conflict-free Ego, this experience can be both creative and restitutive. The immature Ego either never unfolded or, if it had, it remained stunted and fixated. Weaker Egos are enmeshed in the myopic attitudes of others, and by incorporating values of others, they not only subvert their own, but also split their consciousness, depersonalize, and lose a part of themselves.

For example:

> When a loved one dies, and the bereaved person cannot accept the loss, he tries to undo the loss. He may begin to go through rituals to bring the dead one back, he may create legends, or even invest the dead one with magical powers. The mourning of undoing leads to mawkish nostalgia, depression, and severe feelings of unreality.

Loss, death, and conflict are all part of life. And that's the deal! Any good doctor will lose patients, no matter how diligent, or capable he is. An infantry commander knows that in any combat engagement, notwithstanding the valor of his men, he shall lose men—always the price! No matter how much we may love one another, ultimately we must say "until we meet again." In its development, the budding Ego, if it is ever to accept the reality of the deal, must gain its own definition and must belong to its own deep center. At some point, we all must say good-bye to each other. Even in well-aspected relationships, loss is difficult to deal with. This is especially true for children. For them, the loss of a loved one is beyond their comprehension and to help them weather such a storm is a daunting experience.

The body image is the core of the emerging Ego. What one feels about one's body and its body parts, I refer to as the bodily Ego. The feelings associated with one's thoughts form the mental Ego. Feelings that suffuse the body and the mind fuse to create the Ego feeling that holds the Self together. This Ego feeling when withdrawn creates a loss of Ego wholeness, and then depersonalization and derealization ensue. Such Egos are weak and in parts, and they are so divided that they never develop resonant Self-love, or healthy narcissism. If harmony of feelings, thoughts, and actions does not occur, no well-formed Ego boundaries will be defined, and as a consequence, such a person cannot develop a selectivity toward those who influence his behavior. The Ego remains undifferentiated, and is as vulnerable to the outside world, as a turtle on its back lying on a thruway. This is the kind of Ego that becomes caught up in the guilt and shame of others, and resorts to omnipotent delusions and selfish expectations. They become injustice collectors. A poorly differentiated Ego would employ primitive defenses, such as denial and magical undoing, and more readily surrender to the values of others, for they never develop a deep center. The Ego must be sufficiently pristine to decipher the outside world because this data must be presented to the Self to determine *what does Life mean, what can I hope for*, and *what ought I do!*

The meaning of Life must bear a connection to the ultimate concerns of the Self beyond one's psychology and involves its transcendental Self. Is this not what great music and literature seek—that part of ourselves that waits for us over the rainbow? The relationship with oneself must be pure and whole. To develop relatedness to the Other, the Cardinal virtues must meet the Cardinal sins: greed, gluttony, pride, avarice, sloth, anger, and lust. While the Cardinal virtues are directed outward to the other, the Cardinal sins direct the world of the others to its own needs. The Cardinal virtues indicate that people are not God, nor omnipotent; the Cardinal sins satisfy the hedonism of the Self. The fulfillment of the tumescence of the Cardinal sins signifies the hedonistic paradox: the more one lives for oneself, the more unfulfilled one feels. In contrast the fulfillment of the cardinal virtues liberates the Self to its free expressions and choices. Indeed the virtuous are free in their choices, while the licentious remain addicted to their senses.

In social development, the relationship between the Self and the Other takes on the rules of the game, which determines how human beings treat each other. There can be no game without rules, and there can be no social interaction without rules. How could automotive traffic proceed at a busy intersection without the STOP/GO of the traffic lights? What one ought to do requires a decision between what is right and what is wrong. This is a moral duty, and ethics is the discipline applied to this duty. In the emergence of the individual there are two tracts to these rules of morality: one is horizontal across the Earth, and the other vertical, and is upward beyond Earthly boundaries:

1. The *horizontal* one is psychological and is related to the Superego. This is learned, and socially dependent. This social consciousness is a social consensus, and it is the result of what has been taken in (introjected) and assimilated, and
2. The *vertical* one is independent of social consensus, for it arises from the illative faculty of the

mind that seeks universal good in a global consciousness, and it is innate.

As discussed previously, if the majority in a society declares that all people wearing eyeglasses should be imprisoned, the majority rule would be a valid conclusion for the wrong reason. That is social consensus. Conscience would be expressed by that one non-eyeglass wearing Socrates who would say that it would be wrong to imprison eyeglass wearers. His decision would arise out of the inferential injustice of the social consensus. The majority may rule, but they are not always "right."

The well-differentiated Ego would evaluate more clearly those inner appetites of need-want, and would bring about a clearer regulation by moral will. In the more differentiated Ego, there is then a more distinct development of the Superego and a more distinct manifestation of Conscience. The clearer ethical-moral system fortifies the individual to be true to its Self without resorting to affixing the appendages of others, and also avoids the hubris of carnivorous individualism. Once more the individual with more consistent and harmonious values develops those Ego boundaries that are less susceptible to compromise and creates a much more discriminatory person. There are three signs of a well-integrated personality:

1. The ability to hold reality in abeyance for a short time and enjoy the ultimate concerns of What am I to know? What ought I to do? and What do I hope for? In this way, there can be the enjoyment of sports and a sense of humor. Not everything is utilitarian.
2. The ability to discriminate among one's own be-

liefs and attitudes, and yet be open to the thought-feelings of others without surrender of the Self; to be true to one's Self, but open to the world. The Self then has developed an object constancy of itself, and

3. The ability to transfer feelings from the Self to the Other. This transfer can effect values, e.g., celibacy over marriage. Feelings can so be transferred from people to things (linking objects).

The ability to enjoy life in face of its turmoil and mystery, the need to be true to oneself, and the need to be cared for and to care for another completes the personalization of a human being. In this personalization, all human beings join that creative minority of transitional individuals when they choose to face traumatic events either immediately, or through repression. Repression postpones awareness, and when the affects mount into consciousness, there is the opportunity to deal with it all (see Appendix). In contrast, denial is a dead end. Despite the pain of awareness of the trauma, facing its existence is the key for *all* people who want to deal with it in a creative way. The person must first become human and in this process, there is the development of the deep center.

Victor E. Frankl was an Austrian-Jewish psychiatrist who was imprisoned in the dehumanizing experience of the concentration camps at Auschwitz and Dachau during WWII. As a victim/prisoner, he focused not only on survival, but also he became an observer as to what was happening to him and the other victims. In his book *Man's Search for Meaning,* Frankl said that he was "caught up in a mental turmoil which threatened all values." He found himself in a world that no longer recognized "the value of human life and human dignity."

Frankl felt that if he did not struggle against such tyranny, he would lose his self-respect, and he would never know the feeling of being an individual with a mind, personal freedom, and personal value. He became aware that as he felt himself to be only a part of an enormous mass of people in the concentration camp, his "personal ego finally suffered a loss of values," and his existence "descended to the levels of animal life."

When the Ego is confronted with danger to its integrity, the Self must possess a personal inner being and a clear focus as to its outer becoming. Such a transformation from within-out must be carried on the shoulders of personal values. Personal signifies that the knowing, the "oughting to do," and the hoping belong to a particular individual. An Ego overwhelmed by terror or torn by conflict, an Ego too dedicated to survival beyond personal worth, an Ego too much geared to the pleasure of the *now,* cannot be free to maintain its focus on the meaning of life "beyond the survival of the fittest."

In the unfolding sphere of experiencing, there must eventuate a whole Self, which has been clearly differentiated from the Other and from the world of It. This is the differentiated world of Martin Buber's "I, THOU, and IT." Important to note is that the Self can be Self-organizing, almost Self-creating, of its psychology. This capability is necessary to keep things whole, open, related, and novel. Everything in this universe is related and in a resonant connection with its own self-organizing quality. This self-organizing capacity not only renders the universe novel and dynamic, but also imparts the same ineluctable richness to the human being. As the universe needs the freedom of chaotic unity, so too do human beings. Perfection requires the working through of imperfect systems.

The Sphere of Affective Resolution

Affects are feelings that are directed to another, while feelings are subjective states of being and involve the physiological aspects of breathing, blood pressure, pulse rate and sweating. Children who are well integrated are those who can step into the world without an anticipated dread that the sky will fall down upon their heads. These are the children who have resolved their affective relationships with their parents, one way or another. Once they have resolved the ambivalence of dependency upon their parents, these are the children who have internalized the best of their parents. The temperamental interplay between parent and child plays a large role in the affective resolution. For example, a depressive child with a highly excitable mother would not do as well as a depressive child with a sanguine mother. This temperamental fit goes beyond psychology. In any case, what is internalized of the parent becomes an introject and enters by way of the Superego to become incorporated into the social consciousness with its social consensus. Affective resolution completes the person and becomes the signature of personalization.

As mentioned, the conscience with its global quality, is illative and innate. There are those human beings, referred to as transitional people, who are so well self-moving that they are able to intuit right from wrong beyond parochial and social practice. This ability to go beyond consensus is the end process of humanization. Introjection carries with it an affective component that lends the introject a dynamic quality, which is continuously being worked through to make its assimilation whole. In this working-through process, that which belongs to the fabric of the Self becomes part of its quilt, and that which is foreign diminishes the process of both personalization and humanization. With differentiation of the Ego, affects that belong to the Self are distilled from those of the Other. In this way, the focus of the Self is made clear from its deep center, then the within of the Self, the transcendental part, recognizes what is hostile to its integrity, and is then able to treat the Other as it would want to be treated.

In the development of the Self, the analytic and synthetic capabilities of the Ego, suffused with feeling for itself, must maintain a balance between its need for security and pleasure and the demands of the outside world. The imperative of its survival must be weighed against its need to sustain its self-respect. In being open to the needs of others, its own freedom must be protected. Sacrifice for the Other must never take the quality of the self-defeat of masochism. A balance must be maintained among the tri-cornered *sense* of reality, the *cognitive* understanding of reality, and a *relationship* with reality. Only with a clear vision and focus can a person deal with the frustrations in life, its pain, its disenchantments, its disillusionments, and its disappointments. One must maintain a romance with the gift of life. Those non-fulfillments of the Ego ideal must be placed in the perspective of time: the light of some stars we now see left their stations thousands of light years ago, but our small slice of time still has much meaning for us. Life does not insult us with our "failures." Very often we are the culprits. In carnivorous narcissism, it is all "I," and no limits are set. Indeed, experiences can be egregious traps. Accepting limitations may be a beginning of turning a failure into a blessing.

In the concentration camps, Frankl observed that some Jewish prisoners were taken to be "Capos." These Capos were treated as trustees and were given special privileges. They were chosen from the prisoners "who . . . soon became much like the SS men." These Capos must have identified with the aggressors, and their choices must have been reinforced by their exclusive need for survival. Frankl emphasized that some of the Capos fared better in the camp than they had in their own lives. These Capos were persecuted Jews who could still have been demoted.

As has been described, these Capos so split their Egos that they could look upon the world and treat a Bengal tiger as if it were a pussycat. Once a danger to the Self is experienced, and the Ego splits, then its focus is blurred to the tri-cornered reality mentioned previously. To relate to danger would demand a decision to act, and often, to act with conviction can endanger a person. The Capos chose to treat those members with the smell of their nest as enemies to insure their survival. Their evil action reinforced the evil of the SS. Ironically, victims victimized victims.

Ideally, when the Spheres of Experiencing, Differentiation, and Affective Resolution are in harmony, the world is never split. The Self is not bled by the seepage of a split world of a "it's me or them," perspective, a split world in which science makes no room for faith and morality. This seepage of meaning is subtle and is not visible to most people. This seepage drags down passion with its human emblems. Chuenge-tse in the fourth century observed that "Great truths do not take hold of the hearts of the masses." This is very much similar to the New Testament warning that a prophet is without honor in his own land. That creative minority who attempt to bring needed fire to the campsite has always been alone. When the world is split by denials, values are subverted. These few resist these splits. They know that human beings have the means for an expansion of their consciousness to attain their humanization "to love thy brother as thyself." Those who bifurcate the process away from the Other to the exclusiveness of personal success, produce a generation without passion, filled with ennui and apathy.

Here were decent godless people:
Their only movement the asphalt road
And a thousand lost golf balls. (Eliot, 103)[11]

The coming together of these three spheres lend human beings a creative power, which brings his being into becoming. As pointed out, the way of life must first focus on the individual deep center of integrity and truth, and then turn quickly outward to a fellowship with the Other. Then life is not only interpenetrated, but it is also renewed; and only then does this mortal life transcend death.

My idea for this present work took place when I was a neurology resident at Bellevue Hospital. I was entrusted with the care of a former heroin addict who had fallen onto the subway tracks, suffered a cerebral bleeding and went into a coma. He survived with a neurological defect of partial limb paralysis, but he also had given up his heroin addiction. This may have been the result of an involuntary detoxification. Yet he described a vivid dream: he went before a court of three black-robed judges who gave him the choice of death, or if he was to live, he to had relinquish heroin. He chose to live. Trauma became a command for him to return to life.

I do not suggest a utopia, however, but much more I suggest that when people try to live the Cardinal virtues, a way of life is defined, and this arduous passageway leads to a kingdom of goodness, peace, and a prosperity of the spirit. In such a world, the lives of the creative minority teach that civility is twice blessed: he who gives and he who receives. In such a world, when the door of adversity closes, the door of opportunity is opened.

Case Presentations

Case #1 Jim was a tall, good-looking, 25-year-old single man who was always wrapped up in his own feelings and needs. At one point he began to suffer generalized anxiety. One of his major problems was the great difficulty that he experienced in sharing his feelings with anyone. He was "the King," and only what he wanted was his key to improve his wretched existence. Among the things that he wanted was a perfect world and the perfect woman. Thankfully, Jim had a great sense of humor, and was also able to laugh at himself when I had dubbed him "The King of Hearts." He finally met a very beautiful woman who loved him. But she was not perfect—according to him, her teeth were yellow! After much clinical work, he married her.

Unfortunately, during the course of his marriage, disaster struck Jim in the form of a rapidly developing glaucoma that left him blind. Above all, he never despaired, and kept his sense of humor. Across the years, he and I have continued to be good friends. I still call him the King of Hearts, knowing that he has become an angel of goodness and hope for others. His marriage endured, had successful children, and he devoted his life to helping the blind.

Case #2 Emma and her family were caught up in the maelstrom of the Warsaw Ghetto during WWII. She remembered being so hungry that she would secretly steal food from the family cupboard. Her older sister was able to endure the hardships much better than she.

Despite her guilt feelings, she continued her practice of stealing until the family was transferred to a concentration camp where they were separated. One day Emma witnessed her sister being led to one of the gas chambers. Emma became weak. Ironically, when she herself had been taken to the gas chamber, the gas jets were not working. She was spared, but thereafter she remembered that she not only began to function like the guards, but also she became involved only with her own survival.

After her liberation, she found herself in a constant state of numbing depersonalization associated with chronic anorexia. She had become a very strict mother, and was chronically depressed.

Case #3 Rose was a Polish Jew caught up in the nightmare of WWII. Her family had been annihilated by the Nazis. With the help of her Polish Catholic friends, she was passed off as a Catholic, emigrated to France, and lived her life there as a Catholic.

After the War, she emigrated to America, married, and her son became a physician. She remained chic in dress, affable in relatedness, open-minded, gracious, never bitter. After her husband died, she became depressed, but after some help, she was able to live alone and establish social relationships with others.

Case #4 Victor Frankl was not one of my patients, but he demonstrates so much of what I write about. I studied his experience so thoroughly that I could not surrender the opportunity to include his experience in my monograph. As noted, Frankl spent three years in concentration camps. In his book *Man's Search for Meaning,* he stated that he had based his experience in the concentration camps upon this basic premise:

"Our generation is realistic, for we have come to know

man as he really is. After all, man is that being who has invented the gas chambers of Auschwitz; however, he is also that being who has entered those gas chambers upright with the Lord's Prayer or the *Shema Yisrael* on his lips."[12]

From this premise, Frankl maintained a balance in his reaction to this horrific experience. Frankl believed that there was a strong human need to live in choice, to seek meaning in life, and to live in responsible freedom. Sometimes, human beings cut themselves off from the Other, and unknowingly, they do not recognize the damage suffusing themselves. For Frankl, life belonged to much more than mere existence, and he believed that the human future and its becoming were important. He was aware that there existed biological, psychological, and sociological conditions shaping the human capacity "to rise above such conditions and transcend them—a human being is a self-transcending being."

While in the concentration camp, he became "disgusted" with the "trivial things" of mere existence. He would imagine himself giving lectures on the psychology of the concentration camp. Frankl took a clear look at his problems, and felt that they were in his past. He decided to look at them in an objective way. Spinoza's *Ethics* set the tone:

> Emotion, which is suffering, ceases to be suffering as soon as we form a clear and precise picture of it.
>
> (*Affectus, qiu passio est, deince esse passio simulat que eris claram a destinatam formamus ideam*).[13]

In the final analysis, Frankl felt that his experiences taught him that "the salvation of man is through love and in love," and felt that "love is as strong as death." He believed also that love belonged to "the inner self." After all his suffering, he feared nothing except his God. Frankl referred to the concentration camps as "living" laboratories, and "witnessed some of our comrades behave like swine while others behave like saints." One depended on decision, not condition! He gained an unbelievable wisdom: having nothing left, he knew "bliss, be it only for a brief moment," when he thought of "his beloved." He found that in "utter desolation," he could endure the suffering in "an honorable way" through "loving contemplation . . . of his beloved." Then and only then, did he know the meaning of the words: "The Angels are lost in perpetual contemplation of an infinite glory."

Case #5 A thirty-eight-year-old woman lost her husband when he was forty-three years old. He died a slow death of carcinoma of the lung. He left behind three children: a nine-year-old son, a three-year-old daughter, and a-two-year-old son. His untimely death left the family momentarily overwhelmed. I heeded Spinoza's advice in my management of this family: I devised for myself and for the widow "a clear and precise picture" of what happened. I also contacted a financial advisor for the family in order to structure the distribution of the insurance monies, and recommended that no major changes be made.

Repeatedly I emphasized to the mother that the keystone to the entire treatment of her distressed family was *her* affectivity, that is the emotional tempo with which she would respond to all the aspects of her horrific plight. The quality of her relatedness to the children would be the foundation of their response to this devastation that besieged them. I enlisted the help of her extended family, to have them proffer themselves as nuclei for the foundation of healthy identification patterns.

The mother was not only cooperative, but being a devout Catholic and enjoying responsive parents, she had become a consort battleship. Her husband's death brought to life her own warm experiences as a child, as a wife, as a mother, and as a woman. A cat and a dog were added to the family despite the children's awareness of the brief life expectancies of these animals. I had emphasized to the mother that the trauma of her husband's untimely death could be taken as a command to a new hope. This approach was successful for the following reasons:

1. No responses were bitter, and there were no signs of victimization in this family
2. There were no elements of denial, magical rituals, or exaggerated emotions
3. Through the mother's practice of her faith, the children extended their love not only to animals, but also to other children who themselves had lost a parent
4. The affectivity of the mother was always sanguine and showed deep caring for the children.

And to the time of this writing, this family continues to grow in kindness and hope.

Discussion

Although its progression was slow, Jim's loss of sight was a great trauma. He came from a rather solid family and married a loving wife. In therapy he worked on those narcissistic attitudes that could have weakened his Ego. He learned how to create and nurture that deep inner self so crucial to help one stand fast to one's idea of oneself. He had learned to love another, and although blind, he lived his life in a virtuous way. This was also true for the widow who was able to provide the tranquil leadership as the example to be followed. Her strength of resilience came not only from her social structures, mainly her family, but also the nurture from her deep center. By bringing her faith to her children, she strengthened her own faith in the hope that her family would survive and flourish.

Unlike Rose and Dr. Frankl, Emma would not deal with reality beyond her survival. She never developed that deep center of the Self in which the Other is taken to complete the Self. In contrast, Emma not only took care of herself, but unlike Anne Frank, her identification never was completed with her stronger sister. The harrowing trauma of being exposed to non-functional gas jets intensified her desire for survival. Unconsciously, she identified with the Nazis, just as the Capos had done. Although Rose had posed as a Catholic, she always kept the center of herself, and always remained a Jew. She was able to hold the external reality in abeyance. Jim, Rose, Frankl, and the widow made that final choice to be true to their deep center, and consequently their choice was an act of freedom to give to the Other (see Appendix).

For Frankl, meaningfulness in life could be discovered, at least in one of three ways:

1. To perform a good deed, in the way of achievement or accomplishment,
2. To live a value . . . either by experiencing something, such as a work of nature or culture; or by loving someone, i.e., other than oneself, or
3. To endure suffering

By love, Frankl meant the act of sharing the inner most Self, the deep center, with another human being. The spiritual aspect of love enables one to perceive those deeper essential traits, whose potentialities a loved one helps bring into actuality. As for suffering, which often is inescapable, Frankl takes the traumatic experience as "a last chance to actualize the highest value, to fulfill the deepest meaning . . . what matters above all is in the attitude we take toward suffering." C. S. Lewis expresses a similar attitude so necessary to deal with life:

> Even in literature and art, no man who bothers about originality will ever be original: whereas if you simply try to tell the truth (without caring twopence how often it has been told before), you will, nine times out of ten, become more original without ever having noticed it. The principle runs through all life from top to bottom. Give up yourself, and you will find your real self.[14]

Those who are able to assimilate daunting traumas with an attitude of forbearance really become angels unto themselves, for in deepening their inner Self by extending their effort to life things, they become transpersonal and transcendental. At such a time, they bear a resemblance to the transitional beings. In order to experience a meaning to life as Frankl and Lewis have described, there must be an opening of one's inner Ego boundaries, a surrender to permit entrance to the Other. A reciprocal actualization of potential takes place. A simple example of such extended Self would be the starving mother in possession of one boiled potato, peeling the skin for herself, and feeding her two children with its substance. This kind of caring surrender is of the quality of libidinous love.

More than enduring traumatic events, I suggest that a person must move beyond personal suffering with an attitude of humility and with a strong need to bring help to the suffering of the Other. In libidinous love, everyone whom a person has loved becomes hyperfused into an imageless image through which the outpouring of caring focused to the one is inclusive of all.

In this monograph, I have been dealing with human responses to the suffering of loss. Loss can be followed by pain, helplessness, and hopelessness. Loss can be disorienting with a breakdown in space and time as the socio-psychological connections are cut. I have known patients who became so detached and disoriented that they have crashed their automobiles. Loss is traumatic. To cope with loss, there must be a recognition of the reality that a loss has taken place, there must be an acceptance of the suffering that follows. Accepted with patience and meekness, the suffering can be assimilated into the Self for its growth. There are interesting, derivations of the words suffering, patience, and meek:

1. ***suffering,*** from the Latin *sub:* from below and *ferre:* to bear
2. ***patience,*** from the Latin *pati:* to endure, to suffer

As is a deponent verb, it is passive in form, but active in meaning

3. ***meek,*** from the Latin *mucus:* slime, to let slide easily. The meek bear suffering with a smoothness and in an active way.

Interesting words chosen by the collective unconscious. These words convey from the deep, inner Self that for virtue to mature, there must be the need to bear up and to wait in an active way.

I have given reality a tricornered hat:

1. The sense of what one perceives.
2. The knowledge of what one perceives.
3. The relationship to what one perceives.

The word reality is derived from the Latin word, *res;* the thing, or the fact. As recommended, the first step in a traumatic situation is to deal with the descriptive reality that someone or something has been, or is anticipated to be lost. Frankl recognized that he was caught up in a senseless, dehumanizing, destructive experience. In no way did he identify with this inhuman force and chose rather to review the values of his deep Self. He did not want mere survival, so he studied the enemy, and at the same time, he took care of others. He did not become bitter. He stayed in contact with the loss of his loved ones through his love for them. He never surrendered his belief in the goodness of human beings.

Things happen to people on this ship of fools, and we

must deal with these things. When there is self-doubt and self-pity, the Ego boundaries are weakened, the deep center becomes vacuous, and one is then vulnerable. In a vulnerable psychological state of mind, one does not relate center to center with the Other, but in fearful anxiety, the values of the feared one are introjected into the Superego system. A "parasitic" Superego is the result; the values of the feared one then dominate the core of the Deep Self.[15] Differentiation of the self is lost. Center to center relatedness is also diminished when others are blamed for one's plight. Blaming another detracts from the necessary focus that one must have toward trauma: what it means and its consequences.

I have postulated that the Ego functions in three dynamic spheres. When a harmony among these three spheres is achieved, the Ego then exists in time with its own unique history. Its differentiation not only makes it free, but also makes it responsible for its choices. Resolution of affects clarifies love, dependency, and assertiveness. This harmony heightens Ego awareness, and new awareness fosters the insight that love must extend beyond human boundaries. In this harmonious extension, the deep center is born and developed. In this deep center, Conscience keeps its watch over the Superego.

Without the Other, the Self splits (dissociates), projects (paranoid), displaces (phobias), and denies. The experience of reality is then incomplete. Being the most primitive defense, and the most dangerous, denial must be dealt with early. What makes denial so dangerous is its disavowal of the outside world, and its disclaiming of the inner world of the Self. This is also true of the primitive defense of splitting or dissociation. The importance of harmony of the Ego spheres has to do with freeing the Ego to perceive insights about reality and to release affects appropriately to the Self and the Other. For example, in denial of the threat to the Self in traumatic loss, there may follow body image disturbances such as the physical complaints of Anna O. The suffering attendant to loss must end, but the sadness that goes along with having loved and lost must be accepted and experienced. Attention must therefore be given to the immediate demands of the resultant crisis and requires the sacrifice of one's time and one's pleasure.

Generally, in caring for others, one can literally graft one's own Ego to that of the Other. As a consequence, one's own feeling reactions may have to be held in abeyance. Such a delay of affective response is temporary and not comparable to blotting out a feeling.

During an emotional interregnum, one can still feel, compare, know one's needs, and react in an appropriate manner. In such cases, giving fits the meaning of the word sacrifice (the Latin *sacer,* sacred + *facere,* to make holy). The pain of loss is always there, and it is a holy act to give to another through the pangs of one's own pain if only blunted. In some traumatic experiences, there can be a time lag, a latency period, between the time of the traumatic event and the manifested reaction. For example, for young children the death of a parent is a very difficult experience to assimilate. A delay can therefore help to mobilize adequate means to cope with the loss, but once the full impact of the loss occurs, one can expect a regression, especially in children. Regression is not repression. Regression is a return to a former form of adaptation—it is a psychological breather. As pointed out, the reaction to trauma depends not only on the nature of the trauma and the age of occurrence, but also on the *meaning* of the trauma for the person. Denial and repression are not conscious, but repression is a delay factor. Repression offers the Ego time to assimilate what has happened and a way to repair its emotional and social impact.

With any kind of loss, the Ego must gain the insight that life is to be lived and must go on loving and living, despite further dread of loss. Despite the pain of loss, and the reality that all living things are perishable, one must continue to love oneself and others. Once ready to love again, the harmony of the Ego spheres facilitates insight into the meaning of life. We human beings live in a beautiful Universe, and as powerful as the sting of death is, human beings can resurrect themselves over and over, until they can enter the City of Hope. Belonging to each other in sickness and in health contains the human meaning to this life of joy and tumult, to this life of ugliness and beauty. The dialectic must be consumed to create an eternal light.

Indeed, the three spheres of the Ego are dynamic, and once harmonious, the Ego achieves the awareness of the "A-ha," that deep insight of what is real. In this resolute honesty and peace, the life and death of Socrates suggests that a life not examined is a life not worth living. The developing social conscience, the Superego, is the avenue traveled to the within of the Self to generate the balance between pleasure and the price demanded by reality, for there are no short cuts in this valley of tears. On earth we are here not to be happy, but "to pursue happiness." The Conscience displayed by Socrates, as described, goes beyond social consensus and belongs to those transitional creatures who make up the creative minority. Its origin?

These transitional creatures know themselves so completely that they create themselves. They develop a SUPRAEGO. They are self-organizing and self-creating, and do not fall into a carnivorous, narcissistic abyss.

Their reason for living becomes clearer with each honest judgment. They live unafraid. Those who live in dread of loss of life in loving another leave their boundaries susceptible to incorporating the values of those whom they fear. Perhaps the Capos in the concentration camps belonged to this fearful group, possibly as an identification with the aggressor. These are those whom Rado referred to as "parasitic Super-egos," that is containing a foreign body commander, an enemy to one's Ego Ideal and development of a human deep center. Self-appointed victims are those who fall into holes of their own digging, and develop those "parasite Superegos." Divided against themselves, they blame everyone for what they lack.

Frankl sought a supra-meaning to understand "the question of an ultimate meaning of human suffering" that was beyond "the finite intellectual capacities of man."[16] He felt that "man" must not endure more than "the meaning of life." Much more he had to bear his incapacity to grasp its unconditional meaningfulness in rational terms! In his book, *When Bad Things Happen to Good People,* Rabbi Kushner wrote of the loss of his precious fourteen-year-old son to a rare disease. He described how despite this loss he still related to a loving God. Rabbi Kushner accepted that life is not fair, and referring to *JB*, MacLeish's "JOB," he decided to go on living and to create a new life as JOB had done.[17] JB's wife reaffirms that there is no justice in life: "There is only love." Rabbi Kushner did not identify with the Capo types or with the "victims" of the world; rather, he chose to be identified with The Goodness of God "because He is the best part of ourselves." And he concludes:

> . . . that the ability to forgive and the ability to love are the weapons that God has given us to enable us to live

fully, bravely, and meaningfully in this less then perfect world.[18]

Eating without appetite. Sex without love. Beauty without joy. Reason without faith. Life without meaning. Love without suffering. Appetite, love, joy, faith, meaning, suffering are the handmaidens to human biology, but also they are the substance of all ART. Human combinations and permutations of these handmaidens define Life beyond life beyond Art, for they define the human soul.

The traumata of life can become as commands to bring the best of ourselves to the fore for ourselves and for the Other in full dedication of love and sacrifice. True giving has an implacable urgency to be expressed. Frankl reminded us that those who built those gas chambers were of the same species as those who prayed to God en route to the injustice of their deaths.

In the Bible, Job is rewarded with a new life for his having suffered the "arrows of the Lord." Job did face the reality of God's power to give and take away: "the man is born to labor and the bird to fly." Job's life is made whole by his open relationship to God and his recognition that he was made of "clay." Not having "strength of stones nor a flesh of brass," Job finds himself and accepts that "thou wilt bury me into dust again." As Rabbi Kushner pointed out, this suffering of JB's does not give him a new life, as Job had received. JB gains the wisdom not to blame God for a more just universe. JB ceases to seek justice—he and his wife Sarah look within themselves to find that deep center wherein love dwells.

Herbert Howells was an English composer who, on a beautiful holiday, lost his nine-year-old to an acute episode of polio. Howells was "frozen" by his son's death. He worked through his grief by composing a choral work

HYMNUS PARADISI.[19] This work transfigured his grief. The whole range of his emotions, "even ecstasy," was brought to bear to deal with his pain of bereavement. He not only premiered this composition, but almost fifteen years to the date of his son's death, he conducted it. In this work, he put great emphasis on the idea of *lux* (light), and when he needed to bring the work to "an even more intense degree of the work's pervasive radiance," he found it in the sixth movement, "Holy is the True Light":

Holy is the true light, and passing wonderful.
Alleluia
Lending radiance to them that endured in the heat of
the conflict.

Only from a deep center of enduring love, can one "inherit a home of unfading splendor." Sarah says at the end of *JB:*

Blow on the coal of the heart,
The candles in churches are out.
The lights have gone out in the sky.
Blow on the coal of the heart
And we'll see by and by. . . .[20]

To transcend the suffering of the trauma of life, human beings must become whole and distinct as persons. From their experiences, human beings must bring their Selves to the Other. Only in developing such integrity and love, only in such humanization beyond personhood, only then are we ready to light up the stars once more, only then will divine love be experienced. Only at that moment of such radiance will the picture of the Universe be completed.

Indeed suffering human beings must "blow on the coal of the heart." Deaf Beethoven from his deep center gave us a divinelike example of radiance when his inscription on the glorious *Missa Solemnis* read

> *Von Herzen—Möge es wieder—zu Herzen gehn!*
> (From the heart—may it again—go to the heart)

Conclusion

Human beings are very vulnerable creatures. They are confronted with losses very often in their lives. The loss of a parent may be more devastating than the loss of a limb, and yet for some people, this may not be so. When human beings do not attain what they are capable of managing, that is *disappointment.* When they are capable of achievement, but the "system" thwarts them, then they are *disillusioned.* When they have an IQ of 90 and insist on studying theoretical physics, that is *disenchantment.* These unfulfilled expectations can be very traumatic to many people, since they can be experienced as blows to their self-esteem, as putative losses.

In the pluralistic society of the twentieth century, there had emerged a new social-psychic pressure, that of increased specialization. With this inexorable phenomenon, personalization and humanization may be strained to emerge. The humanities stress the whole human being and seek the unity of knowledge and life; and yet science must isolate small aspects of reality and seeks no purpose other than the fulfillment of the Null Hypothesis.[21] This is the essence of the Scientific Method. Science can help to alleviate human suffering, but science cannot bring meaning to such suffering beyond reason.

A harmony of the Ego Spheres of experiencing, differentiation, and affective resolution creates human beings who have awareness of this energy. With time, and through an affective fine-tuning, human beings develop not only a social Super Ego, but also a deep center to the Self, in which the Other is taken to be a crucial part of this Self. In this deep center, the Conscience grows, and has a grasp of the universal human condition: to treat others as they would want to be treated. A clear definition of oneself permits a person to deepen his Self, but never at the expense of the suffering of another!

In closing, I must emphasize that I do not posit a determinism of any kind. I do not believe that life is fixed and dooms human beings. Much more I feel that life is dynamic and self-organizing. In a previous work, *The Swelling Tide,* I wrote of the plasticity and resiliency of the nervous system. I agree with Thomas and Chess that "Temperament is not immutable. . . . Like any, characteristic of the organism, its features can undergo a developmental course that will be significantly altered by environmental circumstances."[22]

In an open system, such as Ilya Prigogine's "dissipated structures,"[23] I wrote in *The Swelling Tide* that chaos arrives at bifurcation point. Supplied with more energy (grace, or information) at such a point of the system, the order of neg-entropy evolves a much more complex system. Without that input, the hegira of disorder/entropy would ensue.

And so it is with the development of human potential, including human response to traumatic events.

Indeed temperament, differentiation of the Ego, the development of a deep center of human values, and family experience are important for the fulfillment of the potential-actual unfolding, but individual personal style carries those tacit, transcendental inclinations that go beyond the concrete, physical, deterministic world of closed systems. This transcendental inclination is self-organizing and dynamic. To be born into the "wrong environment" and the "wrong" initial conditions is not to be without hope. In an open system, when the degrees of freedom shorn of easy assumptions and convenient explanations, are subtracted from human choices, then an individual can be capable of responding to trauma as a command to grow. Either born to the "right" milieu, or to the "wrong" one, human beings can rise above the noise to give direction to the time and chance of Ecclesiastes.

Once trauma is taken as a command to transcend personal suffering, then trauma may have entered into a symbiosis with life, and the stars will shine in the heavens forever. Then we human beings will all be "reconciled among the stars,"[24] world without end!

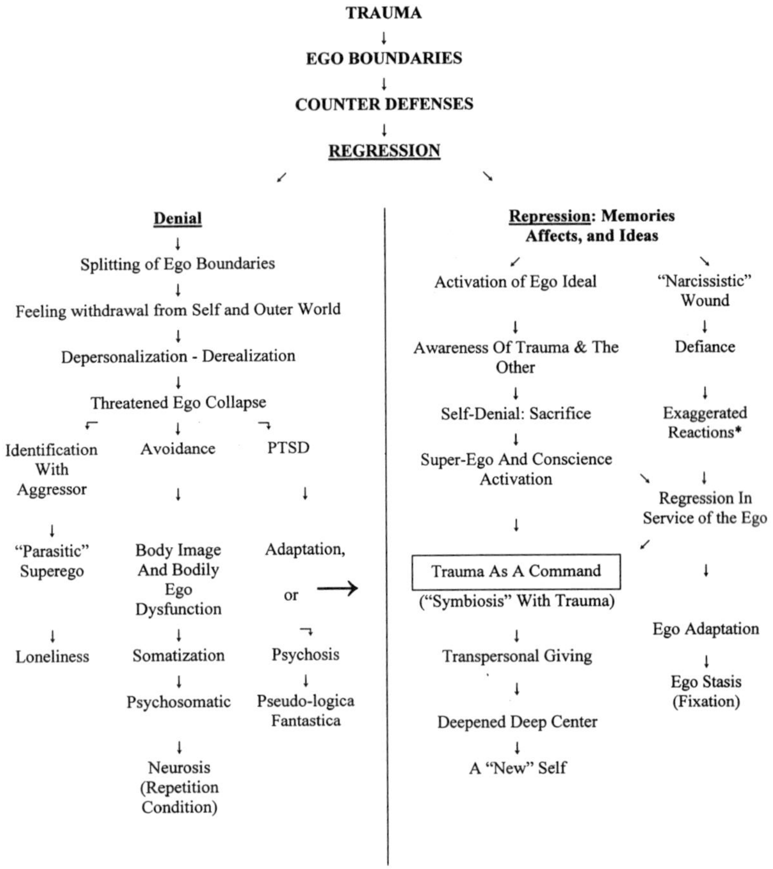

*Exaggerated reactions push affects out of consciousness (repression), not acted out.